Bubbles Bath Bombs and other Bathroom Treats

DIANA PEACOCK

ISBN-13:
978-1530246908

ISBN-10:
1530246903

CONTENTS

THIS BOOK IS A GUIDE

We accept no responsibility for any health or other difficulties
You may accrue having used these recipes.

ALL THESE RECIPES HAVE BEEN USED FOR MANY YEARS ON
NORMAL SKIN TYPES BUT YOUR
SKIN MIGHT BE DIFFERENT

THEREFORE THE RECIPES SHOULD BE USED
AT YOUR OWN RISK

1 INTRODUCTION

In recent years home crafted soaps have become chic and carry with them a chic price tag too! However, the basic ingredients that go into making these toiletries, apart from the oils, are cheap. What's more, making your own soaps, bath bombs and other toiletries is creative, fun and simple.

Another big plus is that you can make concoctions that suit your own skin and hair needs. Most importantly you can leave out unnecessary ingredients like parabens and other preserving ingredients as your products are not going to have to sit in a container on a ship and then on a shelf in a supermarket for weeks on end. In fact, some of the ingredients you use may require you to keep the soap in the fridge!

A few of the shower and bath gels are soap free so even extra sensitive skin can enjoy the benefits of these homemade cleansing products.

Thanks to the joys of the Internet sourcing ingredients is much easier these days. That's not all that helpful to people still without access to the Internet, though. At the end of this book I have included, wherever possible, full contact details including addresses and telephone numbers of suppliers of all the ingredients you will need. Soap and liquid gel bases are sold in both small and large quantities so you won't have to buy a vast amount when you are first starting out.

Once you have mastered the techniques you can go on to make very impressive gifts or even set up a small business. After all, famous high street chains such as Body Shop and Lush started out as home based businesses.

Whether you want to dabble and make a few bath bombs for Christmas or want to have a stand to sell you wares at a local craft fair I am sure you will find, as I do, that you become addicted to making your own soap products and will start dreaming up new recipes to try out on your family and friends.

One final point I will make is that I have tried and tested all of these recipes on my myself and my family. If you have sensitive or problem skin or any such skin disorder you must seek medical advice before using anything new on your skin. If in doubt try a patch test. You should also seek medical advice and follow all safety rules if you are pregnant.

2 KNOWING YOUR ESSENTIAL OILS AND PLANT EXTRACTS

In recent years home crafted soaps have become chic and carry with them a chic price tag too! However, the basic ingredients that go into making these toiletries, apart from the oils, are cheap. What's more, making your own soaps, bath bombs and other toiletries is creative, fun and simple.

Another big plus is that you can make concoctions that suit your own skin and hair needs. Most importantly you can leave out unnecessary ingredients like parabens and other preserving ingredients as your products are not going to have to sit in a container on a ship and then on a shelf in a supermarket for weeks on end. In fact, some of the ingredients you use may require you to keep the soap in the fridge!

A few of the shower and bath gels are soap free so even extra sensitive skin can enjoy the benefits of these homemade cleansing products.

Thanks to the joys of the Internet sourcing ingredients is much easier these days. That's not all that helpful to people still without access to the Internet, though. At the end of this book I have included, wherever possible, full contact details including addresses and telephone numbers of suppliers of all the ingredients you will need. Soap and liquid gel bases are sold in both small and large quantities so you won't have to buy a vast amount when you are first starting out.

Once you have mastered the techniques you can go on to make very impressive gifts or even set up a small business. After all, famous high street chains such as Body Shop and Lush started out as home based businesses.

Whether you want to dabble and make a few bath bombs for Christmas or want to have a stand to sell you wares at a local craft fair I am sure you will find, as I do, that you become addicted to making your own soap products and will start dreaming up new recipes to try out on your family and friends.

One final point I will make is that I have tried and tested all of these recipes on my myself and my family. If you have sensitive or problem skin or any such skin disorder you must seek medical advice before using anything new on your skin. If in doubt try a patch test. You should also seek medical advice and follow all safety rules if you are pregnant.

3 USING 'MELT AND POUR' SOAP BASES

My guess is that this is the real reason you have bought my book! I want to show you that making your own soap is fun, practical and creative. I love planning what I am going to add and I love experimenting with the ingredients and then using them. I have learned that part of the process is getting it wrong as well as getting it right. I would therefore advise that you become a bit of a soap nerd and make notes of ingredients and quantities. I have learned the hard way by repeating mistakes and, even more annoyingly, forgetting what has gone into a soap that has become a big hit with my family.

What are 'melt and pour' soap bases?

Melt and pour soap bases are the easiest way to make soap. They don't use and nasty chemicals and are user friendly.

The base comes in a solid block, often sold in kilo weights through specialised outlets. They can also come in flakes.

They arrive like giant lumps of waxy cheese but clear in colour. Your first task will be to melt the quantity you need in a heatproof bowl over a pan of simmering water or in a microwave. This enables you to add other ingredients such as essential oils, colours, moisturisers and fragrance to make your own personalised soaps and body bars.

The soap bases are reasonably priced and you can get them in different kinds, from basic white opaque to transparent glycerine based soap.

Reputable companies will list the ingredients used in the manufacture of their soap bases. Some are free of the following ingredients: sodium lauryl sulphate, parabens, sodium laureth sulphate and palm oil (the latter being more of an ecological issue). They are made from coconut or rapeseed oil bases instead.

Some are organically made and others have aloe vera, honey based ingredients or plant extracts in the ingredients. They also come in small 500g packs up to trade weights.

Getting Started

What equipment will I need?

- A large pan
- A heatproof bowl that fits inside the pan like a double boiler
- A long handled heatproof spoon
- Some firm plastic moulds (see the section on moulds)
- A hob
- A tea towel to stop you from burning your fingers

Apart from the soap base what other ingredients will I need?

This is a long list as there are many kitchen items you can use plus ones that can be purchased from craft shops and soap making supply outlets. However, I would just concentrate on using what you've got to hand to start with.

Don't be tempted to throw everything into your soap bars. Think about what you want to create before you start and plan your ingredients to match. For a soothing bar, for instance, you could add lavender or chamomile oil and some oatmeal as all are gentle on the skin.

Here is a useful list on ingredients. You won't need all of them so just choose the ones you wish to use:

- Essential oils of your choice
- Fragrances of your choice. You can make your own soap using your favourite perfume rather than spending a fortune on one from the shops.
- Pigments if you wish to colour your soap.
- Salt. Coarse salt can be used as a scrub and fine salt is used to stop the soap from disintegrating.
- Powdered milk makes an excellent soothing emollient additive.
- Oils or butters such as olive oil or shea butter, if you wish to add a moisturising agent. I sometimes add an evening primrose capsule of oil by piercing the gelatine shell and stirring it in (see suggested recipe section).
- Chopped fresh herbs or dried ones.
- Oatmeal. This makes a great additive to soap as you get the skin softening properties of the oats and it is a very gentle exfoliator.
- Desiccated coconut used as a gentle exfoliator
- Ground almonds, again used as a gentle exfoliator
- Loofah particles. These make an excellent addition to exfoliating soaps.
- Various seeds like poppy or sesame to use as gentle exfoliators.
- Ground peach or apricot kernels can be used as a coarser exfoliator.
- Dried flower buds or fruit slices. These can be prepared at

home or purchased.

- Whole or ground spices to fragrance the soaps.
- Plant extracts such as calendula or lavender to add to the effectiveness of the soap. Algae or seaweed extracts and powders can also be added.
- Plant infusions such as rosemary or thyme.
- Lemon or lime juices for freshness and added cleansing.

Colouring your soap

Pigments used in soap and toiletry making come in powder or liquid form. The liquid pigment is the easiest to use. Food colourings can be used but be careful with the amounts used as they can easily stain the skin. Back in the 1970s when 'punk' was literally hitting the streets, a friend of mine used blue food colouring on her hair. All went well until it rained. It didn't come off her skin for ages, much to our amusement!

If you have ever used colours for icing you will know that you have to be careful when adding the colour to the mixture. It is best to use a pipette so that you can control the amount you add. I always wear thin rubber gloves when using the colours as they are very difficult to remove from your fingers, though once mixed into the soap it won't colour your skin at all.

Moulds

When you have finished melting and mixing your soaps you will need to pour the mixture into moulds. You can buy soap moulds of all shapes and sizes. Some have motifs embedded in them and are incredibly fancy. I have to confess I have never bought any!

I wash and keep various plastic cartons such as yoghurt and food pots that have an interesting shape and will withstand heat. I have also used the lidded plastic containers that you get takeaway food in. These are great for making rectangular body soap for use in the shower. Litre sized ice-cream tubs are also useful for making a large cake of soap for you to cut to size as you need it.

4 LET'S MAKE SOAP

1. Get all your ingredients and moulds ready. Fill a large pan with boiling water up to the base of where the heatproof bowl rests. If you are using the microwave then you will need a microwavable bowl.

2. Take the desired amount of soap base. 100g of base makes a 100g bar, it's as simple as that. If the soap base is in a block, chop it into small pieces with a sharp knife and put it in the heatproof/microwavable bowl. If you are melting your soap base in a microwave then it's best to stick to no more than about 300g of soap base.

3. Use a tea towel if necessary to avoid burning your fingers and place the bowl inside the pan. Put the pan on the hob and heat it back up to a simmer. If microwaving, place the bowl in the microwave and set it to high.

4. Use a spoon to help move the soap around so it melts evenly. If using a microwave, use 20 second blasts and keep checking the base. Move it around with the spoon.

5. When the base is completely melted add the other ingredients. Do this quite quickly as the base will start to form a 'skin'. Start with oils or butters, as these take the longest to blend in, and finish with essential oils and fragrances. Remove the soap base from the heat just before adding the essential

oils as they will evaporate quickly is the mixture is too hot. As a guide, when adding fragrance or essential oil to your soap use about 10ml per 500g. Stir gently.

6.   Remove from the heat and carefully pour the melted soap into the moulds.

7.   Allow to cool completely. I sometimes put it in the fridge if the weather is hot. It doesn't seem to affect the food contents so long as everything is covered. If you are adding flower buds, petals, whole spices or other decorations to the soaps, allow the mixture to set slightly or they will sink to the centre.

8. Enjoy!

You may find your finished soap feels a little oily if you have added any moisturising oils or that there is a white layer at the top of the set soap if you have used butters. This is simply a small amount of the moisturising ingredient surfacing while the soap sets. It won't be detrimental to the effectiveness of the soap and will continue to have excellent moisturising properties. These soaps don't lather up as well as a bar that doesn't contain any oil or butter, but they will still clean your body.

5 SOAP RECIPES

All the following recipes make 300g of finished soap. You can use whatever size of mould you like. You can also double the quantities to make a large block of soap that can be cut to size. This is best done with a warm knife. Use any type of 'melt and pour' soap base you prefer.

As for colour, add 1 - 2 drops to a teaspoon before stirring into the soap base with the oils. Add another drop if you like a deeper colour or use a pipette as suggested earlier.

When the soaps have been poured into the moulds you can add extra decoration to the top of the soaps, for instance, a lavender flower or a mint leaf. Allow them to set for about 10 minutes before doing this or it will sink. Leaves may be added as soon as the soap has been poured into the mould then gently pressed down onto the surface.

Cleansing Bars

These soap recipes are good at making you feel clean and fresh, especially after sport or on hot days.

Tea Tree and Mint Soap

Ideal for people with oily skin that needs constant attention. The tea tree gently cleanses and helps clear up spots and break outs.

Added ingredients:

- 1 tablespoon chopped fresh mint leaves.
- 10 drops tea tree oil.

Method:

1.   After melting your soap sprinkle the mint evenly over the surface and gently stir it in.
2.   Remove from the heat if using the hob method and stir in the tea tree oil.
3.   Pour into moulds.

The mint leaves will infuse the soap so leave it to develop for 48 hours before using. The leaves will discolour and turn brown but this won't make any difference to the soap.

Lavender, Thyme and Rosemary Soap

An excellent cleansing and deodorising bar for hot weather or after a vigorous workout. You feel clean after just smelling the soap, let alone using it!

Added ingredients:

- 3 level teaspoons chopped fresh thyme leaves or 1 teaspoon of dried.
- 10 drops lavender oil
- 6 drops rosemary oil

Method:

1.   After melting the soap gently stir in the thyme leaves.
2.   Remove the mixture from the hob and stir in the essential oils.

As in the previous recipe, leave for 48 hours to allow the thyme leaves to infuse the soap.

Cypress and Ginger Soap

This is especially good to use on those cold, wintery days. It not only cleanses but the ginger gets the circulation going again. You can use ginger oil or a little freshly chopped ginger in this recipe.

Added ingredients:

- 10 drops cypress oil
- 5 drops ginger oil or a 1cm cube of fresh grated ginger

Method:

1.   Melt the soap base and, if using fresh ginger, stir in at this point.
2.   Add the cypress oil and stir gently. If using ginger oil add at the same time,
3.   Pour into moulds of your choice and leave to set.

This can be used immediately.

Myrrh and Marjoram Soap

This soothes and cleanses the skin, especially during those cold months when skin can get red and sore.

Added ingredients:

- 1 tablespoon fresh chopped marjoram or 1 teaspoon dried
- 1 tablespoon powdered milk
- 10 drops myrrh oil

Method:

1.   Sprinkle the marjoram and the powdered milk over the soap base as soon as it has melted. I find using a tea strainer helps to evenly distribute the milk powder. Do, however, make sure that the strainer is dry otherwise the milk powder just sticks.
Stir the two ingredients in gently.
2.   Remove from the hob and stir in the myrrh oil.
3.   Pour into the moulds and leave to set.

Allow the marjoram to infuse the soap for 48 hours before using.

Herbal Soap

This truly is the freshest soap around and a popular one during the hot summer. It won't stop you sweating but it really helps with whiffs!

Added ingredients:

- 1 tablespoon very finely chopped parsley (fresh is best for this recipe)
- 5 drops rosemary oil
- 5 drops thyme oil
- 8 drops lavender oil

Method:

1.   When the soap base has melted, gently stir in the chopped parsley.

2.   Remove from the heat and stir in the essential oils.
3.   Pour into the moulds and leave to set.

Allow the parsley to infuse the soap for 36 hours before using.

Moisturising Soaps

There are many ingredients you can add to your soap base to give a moisturising finish. Do remember that most of them will cause a slight reduction in the lathering properties of the soap but they will still cleanse the body.

Rose, Lavender and Shea Butter Bar

Shea butter is really good in soap bars. You need very little to make a difference so it is quite economical to use, too. It's got a strange texture. It is fairly solid until your hands, or anything warm, touches it and then it quickly melts. The combination of lavender and rose soothes and comforts dry skin. If you find rose oil too expensive, use palmarosa oil instead.

Added ingredients:

- 2 level teaspoons shea butter
- 10 drops lavender oil
- 10 drops rose or palmarosa oil

Method

1.   After the soap base has melted stir in the shea butter (Tip - warm the spoon first and the shea butter slips off quite easily.
2.   Remove from the heat and add the essential oils and combine gently with the other ingredients.
3.   Pour into the moulds and leave to set.

This soap can be used immediately.

Oatmeal and Sandalwood Bar

Definitely not just for breakfast, oats soothe and moisturise the skin and the sandalwood is good for dry skins that need a little extra care.

Added ingredients:

- 2 level tablespoons medium oatmeal
- 2 rounded teaspoons powdered milk
- 10 drops sandalwood oil

Method:

1. After melting the soap base carefully sprinkle the oats and powdered milk evenly over the soap and gently stir until it is all incorporated.
2. Remove from the heat and stir in the essential oil
3. Pour into the moulds and leave to set.

Allow to stand for 24 hours before using.

Neroli, Aloe and Olive Oil Soap

This is especially good to help soothe and moisturise the skin after sunbathing.

Added ingredients:

- 1 tablespoon aloe vera gel
- 2 teaspoons olive oil
- 10 drops neroli oil

Method:

1.   After melting the soap base dot the aloe vera gel over the surface and trickle in the olive oil, stirring them both together.
2.   Remove from the heat and stir in the neroli oil.
3.   Pour into moulds and leave to set.

This soap can be used immediately.

Coconut Soap

A wonder for very dry skin. For the coconut cream simply mix 1 tablespoon of powdered coconut milk with 1 tablespoon of warm water.

Added ingredients:

- 3 teaspoons coconut oil
- 1 tablespoon coconut cream
- 10 drops frankincense oil
- 5 drops chamomile oil

Method:

1.   After melting the soap base add the coconut oil and cream and gently stir in.
2.   Remove from the heat and add the essential oil, stirring it in to distribute evenly.
3.   Pour into moulds and leave to set.

This is best left for 24 hours before using.

To give the soap some texture, add a tablespoon of desiccated coconut at the same time as putting in the coconut oil. This makes a mild exfoliator for the skin.

Refreshing Soaps

These will help you wake up in the morning or when you are feeling sluggish and a bit dopey. I find that they also help when you are coming to the end of a bad cold. Somehow they help to get rid of the dregs and make you feel a bit more human.

Lemon and Thyme Soap

Both of these ingredients help with catarrh and clearing your head.

Added ingredients:

- Grated zest of 1 lemon
- 1 teaspoon freshly chopped thyme leaves or 1/2 teaspoon dried
- 5 drops lemon oil
- 8 drops thyme oil

Method:

1.   After melting the soap base gently and evenly add the lemon zest and thyme and stir in.
2.   Remove from the heat and add the essential oils and stir.
3.   Pour into the moulds and leave to set.

Leave for 48 hours to allow the thyme and lemon to infuse the soap.

If you want to add texture you can pare the zest of the lemon thinly away from the pith and chop it into little pieces as coarse as you wish and stir it in with the thyme leaves.

If you have an oily skin add 1 tablespoon of lemon juice when adding the essential oils.

Grapefruit Soap

This a wonderfully mild and yet refreshing soap to use whenever you need refreshing and something to give you that extra zing in the morning.

Added ingredients:

- Grated zest or chopped zest of half a grapefruit
- 1 tablespoon grapefruit juice
- 10 drops grapefruit oil

Method:

1.   After melting the soap base add the zest of the grapefruit and stir in gently.
2.   Remove from the heat and stir in the juice and the essential oil.
3.   Pour into moulds and leave to set.

Allow to infuse for 24 hours before using.

Fresh Lime Soap

This really refreshes the mind and body. Usually associated with summer, I find it's a good one to use in cold weather as it reminds me of summer days. You won't need to add any colour to this as the lime does the job in a very subtle way. However, if you don't do subtle then add a few drops of green or yellow food colouring.

Added ingredients:

- Grated of chopped zest of 2 small limes
- 10 drops of lime oil
- 1 tablespoon lime juice

Method:

1. After melting the soap base sprinkle the zest evenly over the surface and gently stir in.
2. Remove from the heat, add the juice and essential oil and stir in.
3. Pour into moulds and leave to set.

Allow the lime to infuse the soap for 24 hours before use.

Peppermint and Tea Tree Soap

This really wakens you up, especially if you accidentally get it into your eyes, so be careful! It's painful.

Added ingredients:

- 2 teaspoons chopped mint leaves
- 8 drops peppermint oil
- 8 drops tea tree oil

Method

1. After melting the soap base sprinkle the mint leaves over the mixture and gently stir in.
2. Remove from the heat and stir in the essential oils.
3. Pour into moulds and leave to set.

Leave for 48 hours before using to allow the mint leaves to infuse the soap.

Sweet Orange and Bergamot Soap

Even the name sounds divine and exotic! This is a wonderfully fresh and fragrant soap and its smell lasts throughout the day. I suggest that rather than grating the zest you cut it into tiny slithers. This adds a little natural colour and texture to your soap.

Added ingredients:

- 1 tablespoon orange zest
- 10 drops sweet orange oil
- 8 drops bergamot oil

Method:

1. After melting the soap base gently stir in the orange zest.
2. Remove from the heat and stir in the essential oils.
3. Pour into moulds and leave to set.

Leave for 24 hours to allow the orange to infuse the soap.

Soothing Soaps

These not only help to soothe the skin but act on the mind as well, particularly useful during an anxious time or a busy day.

Lavender Soap

A pure lavender soap that soothes yet really cleanses the skin.

Added ingredients:

- 5 lavender flowers - gently remove all the tiny flower parts rather than adding a whole head
- 15 drops lavender oil

Method:

1. After melting the soap base sprinkle the flowers over the surface and gently stir in.

2.   Remove from the heat and add the essential oil.
3.   Pour into moulds and leave to set.

Leave for 48 hours to allow the flowers to infuse the soap.

Oat Milk and Chamomile Soap

This is particularly good for red or irritated skin.

Added ingredients:

- 2 level tablespoons oats
- 4 - 5 tablespoons boiling water
- 15 drops chamomile oil

Method:

1.   Put the oats in a bowl and spoon over the boiling water to soak them. Stir and leave for 2 hours.
2.   Press the oat mixture through a sieve so that much of the liquid is extracted. It is this liquid ('oat milk') that will be added to the soap.
3.   After melting the soap base stir in the oat milk.
4.   Remove from the heat and gently stir in the essential oil.
5.   Pour into moulds and leave to set.

This soap can be used immediately.

Evening Primrose and Melissa Soap

This is great for women going through hormonal changes (and for men, too!). It soothes, calms and moisturises the skin.

Added ingredients:

- 2 high strength evening primrose capsules

- 10 drops melissa oil

Method:

1.   After melting the soap base remove from the heat and stir in the evening primrose and melissa oils.
2.   Pour into moulds and leave to set.

This soap can be used immediately.

Exfoliating Soaps

These soaps are particularly good for getting rid of dead skin cells on the surface of the skin. They boost the circulation too which is known to help counteract cellulite.

Geranium and Loofah Soap

You can buy a small piece of loofah and cut it up to the size you require. Remember, it is a particularly coarse exfoliator so it wise to start with very small pieces. The olive oil will help moisturise the skin.

Added ingredients:

- 2 teaspoons olive oil
- About 1 tablespoon loofah pieces
- 10 drops geranium oil

Method:

1.   After melting the soap base add the olive oil and loofah pieces and remove from the heat. Stir in gently.
2.   Add the geranium oil and stir to distribute.
3.   Pour into moulds and leave to set.

This soap can be used immediately.

Orange, Almond and Apricot Kernel Soap

A real circulation booster when massaged into wet skin.

Added ingredients:

- 1 level tablespoon ground apricot or peach kernels
- 2 teaspoons sweet almond oil
- 15 drops sweet orange essential oil

Method:

1.   After melting the soap base sprinkle the ground kernels evenly over the surface and sprinkle on the almond oil. Stir in to combine evenly.
2.   Remove from the heat and stir in the orange oil.
3.   Pour into moulds and leave to set.

This soap can be used immediately.

Sea Salt and Ginger Scrub Bar

This is especially good during cold winter months as it boosts the system and gets rid of old skin cells that lurk under winter clothes.

Added ingredients:

- 2 level tablespoons coarse sea salt
- 1 teaspoon sunflower, peach nut or rapeseed oil
- 10 drops ginger essential oil

Method:

1.   After melting the soap base stir in the sea salt to evenly

distribute it.

2.   Remove from the heat and add the oil and essential oil. Stir in gently.

3.   Pour into moulds and leave to set.

This can be used immediately.

6 BATH BOMBS, MILKS, SALTS AND PARCELS

Remember those square shaped bath salts wrapped in silver in a gift box that you used to give to your grandmother every Christmas? Bath salts have come a long way since then. Now they come in all shapes, sizes, colours and smells, with even the odd bit of foliage and sparkle thrown in for good measure.

Granny will still be pleased but even more delighted as these ones have had thought, and even perhaps her favourite fragrance, added to them.

Bath Bombs

I have a confession....I am addicted to bath bombs. My family calls it my vice. I have spent a fortune on them and they are always on my Christmas present list.

They are great fun, smell divine and leave your body feeling soft and smelling fragrant. The fizzing ones are good if you experience muscle tension as they help soothe you and relax the muscles.

So, given my expensive habit, I had to start making my own. The basic ingredients are really quite inexpensive and imagination is free. A good idea is to get inspiration from shops specialising in these types of 'luscious' things.

You may find it quite tricky at first but keep on trying. The ingredients won't be wasted as you can still use them - just don't give the first batch away as gifts!

I found the hardest bit to master was keeping it moist whilst I was making it.

The main thing I found difficult was using the sprayer. This is an essential part of the process; too much water in the sprayer makes them fizz and expand and then they won't work in the bath, too little makes the mixture harden so you can't use it.

Use cold boiled water or distilled witch hazel to spray on the mixture. Witch hazel is more expensive but doesn't make the mixture fizz or harden as quickly.

Specialist outlets sell a variety of moulds of differing shapes and sizes that make your finished bombs look professional. The round ones comes in halves which you fill and put together and they are particularly reminiscent of shop bought 'bombs'.

However, you could always experiment. Using small plastic containers such as yoghurt pots will be ideal. As the mixture isn't hot when you put it in you have more choice than you have when making soap. I've made them in those silicone cupcake cases that you can buy.

The Basic Method Of Making A Bath Bomb

Utensils:

- A large mixing bowl to mix the dry ingredients together
- A hand water sprayer containing cold boiled water or witch hazel
- Scales to measure the ingredients
- A long handled spoon to mix larger amounts
- A fine sieve
- Moulds

Ingredients:

Once you become more confident in handling the mixture you can vary the amounts used but the quantities below will make 2 large or 3 medium sized bombs.

- 50g citric acid - granular is easiest to use at first but the powdered gives a more professional finish once you get used to it.
- 150g bicarbonate of soda.
- About 5ml fragrance and/or essential oils of your choice.
- Colour. Use liquid food, toiletry grade or powdered.

You can add flower petals, specially made glitter, powdered milks or cocoa butter to make your bombs that little bit more exciting (see the recipe section).

Method:

1.   Make sure the mixing bowl and spoon are completely dry. Put the citric acid and bicarbonate of soda together into the bowl using the sieve to get rid of any large clumps.

2.   Stir well so the two ingredients are evenly mixed.

3.   Use a dropper to add small amounts of the chosen colour or sprinkle evenly if you are using powdered colour. Remember less is ALWAYS best with the colour - you can always add more. Stir it in quickly as you add it until you get the correct depth of colour.

4.   Sprinkle in the fragrance of your choice or add essential oils. Both can be added if you wish to give a fuller fragrance. Stir in quickly as you add it to distribute it evenly.

5.   Stir in any other ingredients you may be using at this stage, unless otherwise stated in the recipes.

6.   Now use your hands to bring the mixture together. With practice you will get to know how it should feel. It's for this reason I don't use rubber or plastic gloves to do this but you can if you prefer.

Press the mixture firmly together with your hands and use your water spray to spray a small amount of cold boiled water or distilled witch hazel onto the mixture as you do so. Work quickly and press the mixture into the moulds. If you are using a round traditional bomb mould, press the mixture into one half until it is slightly proud of the mould edge by a millimetre or two as this bit will adhere to the other half. Do the same to the other mould half and then press them together firmly. Clip the two halves together for 20 minutes until they have set. When you unclip the mould the bomb should come out easily. If you are using other moulds simply press the mixture in and leave it to set, then tip it upside down to remove the bomb.

For the cupcake shaped bombs I use the silicone cupcake tray to make them and then transfer them to individual paper cases once they have set. I decorate them using a plain white soap base (with added colour) and various decorations.

To make bubbly bath bombs mix 50g of sodium lauryl sulphate (SLS) noodles to the dry ingredients. These are tiny pieces of soapy granules similar to the colourful hundreds and thousands you put on top of cakes. They create the bubble in many toiletries. You can purchase them from soap and toiletry outlets. You can also add them to bath milks and salts for a bit of bubble.

Lavender Fizz

A soothing one to relax in.

Method:

Add 15 drops of essential oil and about 8 lavender heads. Remove the tiny flowers from the stem and stir in after adding the colour and fragrance. Add a few drops of violet food or toiletry colour if you wish.

Snowball

This is a wonderful winter fizz bomb, perfect for the Christmas stocking.

Method:

Add 10 drops of ginger oil and 8 drops of black pepper oil. 2 tablespoons of powdered milk stirred into the dry ingredients will give a smooth, silky finish to this bomb. Leave it without colour so it lives up to its name. However, you can use whatever fragrance you like!

Floral Bombs

Method:

To make floral bomb choose a single note fragrance like rose or honeysuckle, add about 5ml to the dry ingredients and stir well.

Add flower petals or tiny buds and colours to match the flower chosen when you have added all the other ingredients.

Vanilla Skin Softening Bomb

Method:

Add 1 teaspoon of grated cocoa butter to the dry ingredients and stir well. Add 10 drops of vanilla fragrance to the mixture.

Bedtime Bomb

Method:

Add 2 tablespoons of powdered milk to the dry ingredients and stir well.

Add 8 drops of lavender, 8 drops of clary sage and 10 drops of chamomile oil and stir in.

Party Bomb

Here's one that's sure to get you in the party mood

Method:

Add a tip of a teaspoon of glitter to the dry ingredients and 8 drops of lemon oil and 8 drops of grapefruit oil and stir well.

Bath Salts

Bath salts are very easy to make and don't have the fuss of pressing and forming them into moulds but they can be made fizzy or bubbly in just the same way. Store them in airtight jars and they will keep for months.

The Basic Method For Bath Salts

To make about 400g you will the same utensils as for bath bombs but you won't need any moulds, just a jar with a secure lid that can easily be removed and replaced throughout use.

For Plain Bath Salts

Ingredients:

- 100g Epsom salts
- 300g extra coarse sea salt
- 1 - 10ml of fragrance or essential oils
- Colours if you wish, as for bath bombs

Method:

1. Mix the dry ingredients together in a bowl.
2. Stir in the fragrance or oils.
3. Add the colour gradually, stirring in quickly.
4. Transfer to the storage jar.

For Basic Lavender Bath Salts

As per the previous recipe but instead of adding the colour, add lavender flower heads before transferring to the storage jar.

For Fizzy Bath Salts

Ingredients:

- 100g Epsom salts
- 200g extra coarse sea salt
- 50g bicarbonate of soda
- 50g granular citric acid
- Fragrance and colour

Method:

1. Mix the bicarbonate of soda with the citric acid.
2. Mix all the dry ingredients together in a bowl.
3. Add the fragrance and colour.
4. Transfer to the storage jar.

For Bubbly Bath Salts

Ingredients:

- 100g Epsom salts
- 200g extra coarse sea salt
- 100g SLS noodles
- Fragrance and colour

Method:

1. Mix all the dry ingredients together in a bowl.
2. Add the fragrance and colour.
3. Transfer to the storage jar.

Bath Milks

Somehow these always sound more exclusive to me than bath salts - it must be the association with Cleopatra! The addition of powdered milk, cornstarch and cocoa butter give them a luxurious sensation and soften the skin.

Basic Method For Bath Milk

Ingredients:

- 120g coarse sea salt
- 35g Epsom salts
- 10g cocoa butter, grated
- 2 level tablespoons dried milk (goats milk or coconut milk are excellent for this)
- 10g cornstarch
- 10ml fragrance and/or essential oil

Method:

1. Mix the sea salt, Epsom salts and milk powder together in a mixing bowl.
2. Stir in the cocoa butter and mix well.
3. Put the cornstarch into a small bowl and add the oil or fragrance or a combination of both. Mix thoroughly and the cornstarch will absorb the liquid part of this ingredient so it can be easily stirred into the other dry ingredients.
4. Stir into the other mixture and store in glass jars with well fitted lids.

Have fun making your own 'potions'. It is amazing how addicted you become to dreaming up ideas.

Here are a few of my favourites. You can use any of the basic recipes above for these.

Ready For Anything

Great for waking up the system before a party or just to revive you.

Method:

Add to the basic mixture:
- 8 drops sweet orange essential oil
- 8 drops lemon oil or fragrance
- 8 drops lime oil or fragrance
- 8 drops ylang ylang

Feel Good

To uplift your mood and give you the confidence boost you occasionally need.

Method:

Add to the basic mixture:
- 8 drops jasmine oil
- 8 drops geranium oil
- 8 drops clary sage
- A few drops of rose fragrance

Bedtime Bath Soak

The milky mixture is best for this soothing soak.

Method:

Add to the basic mixture:
- 8 drops lavender oil
- 8 drops neroli oil
- 8 drops melissa oil
- 5 drops clary sage

Get Clean Quick

This is a good one when you are all sweaty after sport or working in hot temperatures. The fizzy bath salts mixture goes well with it.

Method:

Add to the basic mixture:
- 8 drops lemon oil
- 8 drops lavender oil
- 8 drops rosemary oil
- A teaspoon thyme leaves or 5 drops oil if you prefer

7 SHAMPOOS AND HAIR AND SCALP CLEANSER

Time for another confession - I am also a shampoo junkie. I colour my hair regularly so I buy one kind of shampoo for coloured hair, another because my hair has a tendency to frizziness, yet another one because I like my hair to shine, one to clean my scalp and finally one when it is feeling dry and coarse.

I must be a dream customer because I also tend to buy the matching conditioner as well and end up paying a fortune, not to mention the extension needed for the bathroom and all the additional shelving and cabinets in which to store all the bottles!

So you can see that making my own was eventually the only option to keep my bank account happy. It is definitely cheaper and you can adapt your shampoo to the condition of your hair which will change depending on environment, health, stress levels and lifestyle changes. Anyhow, it's great fun experimenting with different ingredients to see what works for you.

Soapnuts

IF YOU HAVE SENSITIVE SKIN DO NOT USE SOAPNUTS

I have only recently become a convert to this very unusual, natural soap product. Soapnuts can be used for cleaning the body, hair, clothes and furniture very effectively. They are actually the dried husk of the soap berry nut and they have been used for hundreds of years in Asia to clean everything and everyone, from washing clothes to shampoo. Another bonus is that they have an almost endless shelf life. The other very positive aspect to using soapnuts is their impact, or rather lack of it, on the environment as they are 100% biodegradable.

As the properties of these nuts are mild and virtually non-reactive to the skin they are particularly good for cleansing the hair and scalp of people with psoriasis or eczema. Due to their anti-bacterial and anti-fungal properties they are also excellent for anyone with a skin condition.

Surely, you say, there must be a downside. Well the one disadvantage with using soapnuts that I have found is that they have an acidic smell. Don't let that put you off, though. As soon as you add your choice of essential oils this fades.

On contact with water, soapnut shells release saponin, a natural surfactant that breaks down the surface tension between water and grease, enabling the grease to be washed away. I'm afraid soapnuts haven't made it on to supermarket shelves yet but you should be able to find them in specialist health outlets and, of course, they can be purchased quite easily from internet sites.

Using Soapnuts To Make Shampoo

Have a large sterile plastic or glass container ready with a secure lid.

Method:

1. Add about 20 pieces of soapnut shells to 1.5 litres of hot

water. Bring to the boil and continue to boil for 30 minutes.

2.   Top up with a little boiling water from time to time. Allow the liquid to cool before lifting the nuts out. These can be reused in your clothes washing.

3.   Pour the cooled liquid into the container and secure the lid.

You can now use this to make up your shampoo recipes. It makes about 6 shampoos worth of base as you will use more to cover your hair than normal shampoo.

I make up about 30 - 50ml at a time. This suffices for one dose and you can add different ingredients depending on the condition of your hair and your personal preference. Although the soapnuts themselves have a long shelf life the made up solution will not so you will need to store this for up to 4 weeks in the fridge or a cool dark place.

As with any product DO NOT GET THE LIQUID IN YOUR EYES! I DID AND IT HURTS LIKE MAD. IF YOU DO RINSE YOUR EYES WITH COLD WATER IMMEDIATELY AND SEEK MEDICAL ATTENTION.

To thicken the hair washes that I make I mix about 25ml of the hair wash with a dessert spoon of thick natural yogurt. This helps to thicken the application and has a wonderful softening effect on my hair. It rinses out fully without leaving a greasy film on the hair.

To use, wet your hair as normal then pour over the soapnut mixture and massage into the scalp and hair, making sure it goes nowhere near your eyes. Leave it for a few minutes and then rinse away as with normal shampoo. This will not create much in the way of suds but will clean your hair and scalp very efficiently.

Have a towel ready to wipe any mixture away from your eyes.

- Add 5 - 8 drops of tea tree essential oil to really clean away scalp debris and help with dandruff. Leave on for 5 minutes.
- Add 8 drops of lavender essential oil to soothe and clean itchy or red scalps. Leave on for 5 minutes and rinse as normal.
- Add 8 drops of lemon essential oil and 2 teaspoons of lemon juice to help with oily hair and keep it feeling light and 'swingy'. This is also good to give shine and softness to blonde hair. Leave it on for 8 - 10 minutes.
- Add 8 drops of rosemary oil and 2 tablespoons of rosemary infusion.
- Simply boil 1 teaspoon of rosemary leaves in 100ml of water in a small pan or microwave. Keep it boiling for 2 minutes then allow everything to cool together before straining the liquid into a sterile bottle or jar. Use within 14 days. This makes dark hair shine and enhances the colour. It is also very good for the scalp. Leave it on for 10 minutes.
- Add 8 drops of ylang ylang essential oil to balance the scalp if it is over oily or dry. It makes the hair smell wonderful too.

Soapwort

This is another completely natural hair cleansing ingredient. Soapwort, like soapnuts, contains saponin, but this is grown in the United Kingdom. It is safe to use on the skin and is 100% biodegradable. Again it doesn't have a great lathering ability but this doesn't reflect on the finished result. The dried soapwort root can be purchased from some health food stores and from internet suppliers or you could grow your own.

The shampoo base is made in a similar way to the one in the soapnuts section. This recipe will make about 6 doses of shampoo.

Ingredients:

- 2 level tablespoons of dried soapwort root
- 1 litre of hot water

Method:

1.   Bring the water and soapwort root to the boil then cover and simmer for 25 minutes.
2.   Allow everything to cool together then strain the liquid into sterile lidded bottles or jars
3.   Store in the fridge and it will keep for 14 days.

The above recipes can all be used with this shampoo base.

Try these as well with the soapwort mixture.

Put 3 chamomile teabags in 100ml of boiling water and simmer for 10 minutes. Allow it to cool with the tea bags still in the water. Squeeze the liquid out of the teabags and discard. Add 10 drops of chamomile essential oil. Combine this with 30ml of the soap base. Wet your hair as normal and squeeze out any excess water. Apply the shampoo mixture and massage into the hair and scalp. Leave for 10 - 15 minutes then rinse out. This is particularly good for fine hair and blondes as it adds golden highlights and shine.

For a healthy scalp and soft clean hair mix together 1 teaspoon of rosemary leaves, 6 lavender flower heads and 1 tablespoon of young nettle leaves. Chop everything together and put in a small pan with 100ml of water. bring to the boil then simmer for 10 minutes. Watch the pan doesn't dry up. Add a little more boiling water in necessary. Allow everything to cool together then strain the liquid into a bottle or jar. Use within 2 weeks and store in the fridge.

Use 1 tablespoon of this mixture with 8 drops of lavender oil and

30ml of shampoo base. Wet the hair as normal and squeeze out excess moisture. Apply the shampoo and massage into the scalp. Leave for 5 minutes before rinsing out.

Other Ways Of Making Your Own Shampoo

As with the melt and pour soap bases you can also purchase melt and pour shampoo bases. These can be mixed with your own ingredients to make your own concoctions suitable for you and your family.

They are melted in the same way as soap, either over a double boiler or in a microwave for a few seconds at a time. Then add your own ingredients to make a bar. Pour it into a simple mould and allow it to set.

8 HAIR RINSES CONDITIONERS AND MASKS

Conditioning your hair can be an expensive affair especially if, like me, your hair condition changes quite regularly. I find the best way to condition my hair is to not use shampoo for about 5 days. This gives the natural oils a chance to recover. My hair feels softer and somehow remains cleaner and shinier for longer. When I do finally wash my hair I tend to use a rosemary based shampoo to clean and freshen and finish with cold water to smooth down the cuticles.

But sometimes more conditioning is necessary, especially after a beach holiday or during cold windy weather, which always seems to dry my hair. Times like these call for a conditioning mask.

Here are some of my favourite tried and tested hair conditioners and rinses that are quick and quite inexpensive.

Hair Rinses

These are great as a light conditioning treatment that helps smooth down the cuticles on the hair and they make a real difference to the hair, making it look and feel healthy.

They are easy to prepare and most of the ingredients may already be in your kitchen.

Plain ice cold water makes a simple yet effective frizz tamer and cuticle smoothing final rinse. It also helps keep oil at bay. The trouble is it is very cold but worth it in the end!

Vinegar Based Rinses

Vinegar is an excellent ingredient as it makes the hair shine. Don't worry about the smell! It may whiff like a fish and chip shop at first but I promise you, when dry the smell disappears. Don't be tempted to rinse the vinegar away as the hair benefits from it being left in.

For All Hair Types And Shades

Method:

Add 1 tablespoon of cider vinegar and the juice of 1 lemon to 500ml of cold water. After shampooing and rinsing out the suds completely, pour the liquid over the hair, coating every strand.

For Drier Hair Types

Method:

Add 1 tablespoon of malt vinegar to 500ml of cool water. Whisk in 5 drops of olive oil just before you are ready to pour the water over the hair. Massage it into the scalp a little before towel drying.

For Adding Highlights To Brown And Red Hair

Method:

Add 1 tablespoon of red wine vinegar to 500ml of cold water and pour over the hair after rinsing out the shampoo.

Beer

This is good for adding shine and body to your hair - honest! It plumps up the hair so a word of advice - avoid this as I have to do if you have thick hair. I tried it once and looked as though I had a wig on!

Any beer will do so don't worry too much about staying loyal to your favourite pint. It isn't the alcohol that conditions the hair, it is the other ingredients, so using inexpensive beer is just as good for the hair.

Herbal Hair Rinses

These can be made using dried herbs, though fresh ones will give you the best and most intense results.

They should be applied after washing your hair as a final rinse. Pour them over your head and massage into the hair and scalp with the fingertips and squeeze out the excess moisture before towel drying the hair.

For Dark Hair

Method:

Chop 2 tablespoons of fresh rosemary leaves and put them into a jug. Pour 350ml of boiling water over them and stir and macerate the leaves. Allow it to go completely cold. Strain the liquid and pour over the hair.

For Blondes

Method:

Steep 3 chamomile tea bags in 350ml of boiling water and allow to go cold before squeezing out the liquid from the bags. Add 1 tablespoon of lemon juice and pour through the hair. If you blow dry your hair after using this it will intensify the effect.

For A Healthy Scalp

Method:

Add 1 tablespoon of thyme leaves to a jug and pour over 350ml of boiling water. Stir and bash the leaves to get the oil out. Allow it to cool then strain the liquid. Add 5 - 8 drops of tea tree essential oil and pour over the hair. Massage into the hair and scalp for 1 minute. This has the added benefit of keeping head lice away and is therefore particularly useful when you have children.

For Mature Hair

Method:
Add 10 drops of frankincense essential oil to 400ml of warm water and massage into the hair and scalp. Leave in for best results without rinsing out. Your hair will smell wonderful.

Conditioning Treatments

Usually these are best used before shampooing the hair as they have a large amount of debris that is best washed away with more than just water. I find that using one of the following before washing, then a rinse after shampooing, leaves my hair in excellent condition. These only need to be used once a week for the best results.

Banana Conditioner

This is ideal for normal to dry hair that needs extra conditioning. The yogurt seems to help the scalp get rid of dead skin cells.

Method:

Mash 1 large banana and mix it with a teaspoon of clear runny honey.

Stir in 2 good tablespoons of natural yogurt. Apply to damp hair and massage into the hair and scalp. Put on a plastic shower cap or wrap in a warm towel or cling film and leave for as long as you can, preferably where nobody can see you!

Avocado Conditioner

This is my favourite for frizzy dry hair.

Method:

Mash a medium sized avocado with an egg yolk and 8 drops of geranium essential oil. Apply to the hair and scalp, massaging in gently but firmly. Wrap the head as before and leave for at least 30 minutes.

Olive Oil And Honey Conditioner

This is a moisturising conditioner but it's quite light. It gives shine and softness to all hair types. You should use light olive oil as the extra virgin variety can be a little cloying on the hair. You might find this treatment a little inconvenient if you want to create a look, as it can coat the hair, especially if you use too much olive oil, but after a few days you will see a real difference in your hair quality.

Method:

Mix 1 tablespoon of olive oil, 1 tablespoon of lemon juice and 1 tablespoon of clear runny honey into a bowel. Heat for a few seconds in a microwave or over a pan of hot water. Apply to damp hair and massage into the hair and scalp. Wrap in a warm towel and leave for 15 minutes before rinsing and shampooing.

Mayonnaise

Don't put it all on your eggs! This really is an amazing conditioner and it contains all the ingredients that are good for your hair.

Method:

Just massage 2 tablespoons (no more or it is difficult to shampoo away) into the hair and then smooth your hair down. Wrap your head in a towel or cling film. Leave for at least an hour before washing away.

Cucumber Conditioner

This is a treatment for oily to normal hair. Hair is left soft and shiny.

Method:

Peel half a cucumber and puree it in the food processor or mash it well with a fork. Add 1 whole egg and 2 teaspoons of sunflower oil and mix it together. Apply to damp hair. Wrap the head in cling film or a plastic shower cap and leave for 20 - 30 minutes.

Light Conditioner

This can be used after shampooing if your hair is a touch dry, but rinse out well with warm water.

Method:

Whisk half a teaspoon of olive oil into a whole egg. Beat in 200ml of tepid water, Pour over the hair and massage into the strands, avoiding the scalp if your hair has a tendency to be oily. Leave for 2 minutes before rinsing thoroughly.

Masks

Do you remember girly nights in all sitting around with face masks and hair masks? Well, here's the ideal way to recreate those fun times.

These conditioning masks are thicker and oilier than conditioners and will need to be left on your hair for at least an hour. Wrap your head in cling film to keep in the heat for best results.

Milk And Honey Mask

Actually is isn't really milk but yogurt that is used in this treatment.

Method:

Mix 3 tablespoons of natural yogurt with 1 egg yolk and 1 tablespoon of clear runny honey. Beat in 1 teaspoon of sunflower or jojoba oil and 8 drops of lavender essential oil. Apply to the hair in a thick layer, making sure it is all coated and leave for a few hours.

Coconut Treatment Mask

This is good for thick, coarse dry hair and uses creamed coconut and coconut oil. Both can be purchased in shops quite easily.

Method:

Put 20g of creamed coconut and 1 teaspoon of coconut oil in a bowl over a pan of hot water. They will melt together quite quickly. Stir in 8 drops of lavender oil to soothe the scalp and, if you are over 40, try 8 drops of frankincense essential oil. This is great for mature hair. Beat in 1 egg yolk. Apply to dry hair, massaging it into the strands. Wrap the head and leave for at least 2 hours.

Coconut oil can be applied to dry ends of the hair if you have an oily scalp. Warm a small amount about the size of a penny in your hands until it melts and apply it to the ends of your hair. Comb through and leave for a few hours. Wash out with shampoo and condition as you wish.

9 SHOWER AND BATH GELS

There is nothing more pleasant than getting into a hot bath and just wallowing in the warmth of the water, or going under the shower and using a gel that soothes or awakens the senses. But add to that the pleasure of using products that you have made yourself and what could be better for you and your purse.

Shower and bath gels can be made from scratch with easily sourced ingredients or you can purchase shower and bath gel bases in the same way as the melt and pour soap bases and usually from the same place. These come in various types ranging from basic bases to organic ones. They should specify whether they contain ingredients that may cause irritation to some people, like parabens or sodium lauryl sulphate.

The bases are often concentrated and need diluting with some cooled boiled water before adding your other ingredients. If you are using decoctions that are already liquid based take this into consideration when diluting your bases. The company you purchase these bases from will tell you the dilution ratios as they differ greatly. You can use them in a concentrated form if you wish and just use less but always apply it to a wet sponge, flannel or whatever you like to use in the shower before applying it to your body. Diluting the concentrate bases also makes it easier to pour, especially in the bath.

There are some shower gels you can make completely from your own ingredients. They are good for sensitive skins or just when your skin needs extra care.

The following recipe is a soapless cleanser that is very mild but still works well to clean the skin.

Soapless Shower Gel

You will need a sterile jug and a bottle or container with a secure lid. This way the shower gel will keep for about 2 weeks. It doesn't lather up and is, therefore, a bit disappointing at first but it still cleanses the body well. I've found it best to wet the skin in the shower then turn the shower off while you apply the gel, massaging it in with your flannel or sponge before rinsing it off completely.

Ingredients:

- 300ml cooled boiled water
- 1 teaspoon cornflour
- 2 tablespoons glycerine
- 1 teaspoon caster sugar
- 2 teaspoons sunflower, sweet almond or jojoba oil
- 3 tablespoons aloe vera gel
- 20 drops lavender oil

Method:

1. Mix the cornflour with a little of the cooled boiled water and stir in the rest of the water in the sterile jug.
2. Stir in all the other ingredients gradually, one at a time. Don't add the lavender oil just yet.
3. Pour the shower gel into the bottle and add the lavender oil. Secure the lid and give everything a good shake.

4.   It is now ready to use. Every time you use the shower gel give it a good shake beforehand to mix up the ingredients.

Soap Nut Body Wash

A body wash can be made in the same way as the shampoo base using soap nuts. The saponin liquid from the soap nuts can be thickened with guar gum, this is widely available to buy from online retailers. Thickening the liquid means you don't waste any down the drain.
Use 1 tsp guar gum to 250ml of soap nut liquid and whisk it in when you are adding the essential oils.

Ingredients:

For a concentrated soap nut liquid.
25 soap nut shells to 1.2 litres water

Method:

1.   Place the soap nuts in a large pan as the mixture froths up when boiling, Boil the soap nuts for about 30 minutes in the water, topping up the water with freshly boiled water, use about 100 ml, after about 20 minutes. Watch for the mixture boiling up with the froth.
2.   Allow the liquid to cool before removing the soap nuts. Reuse these in your laundry. They will be good for at least 2 loads.
3.   Add 1 tsp guar gum to every 250 ml whisking in well. The liquid will froth, but this will settle down after awhile.
4.   Pour into bottles and add your favourite essential oil mixture and a few drops of almond, wheatgerm, evening primrose or avocado oil for a little softening and moisturising property of the wash.
5.   Always shake the bottle well prior to using.

The shelf life of the product isn't as long as shop bought body wash so keep in a cool dark place or use within 2 weeks.

Using Ready Made Shower And Bath Gel Bases

These are bases that are highly concentrated and can be used to make up your own recipes quite easily or can be used without perfume or colour for very sensitive skin. They are readily available from specialist outlets but not as easy to find on the high street.

After the initial dilution with cooled boiled water you can add many other ingredients to make showering a pleasurable and 'skin kind' experience. With clever use of essential oils you can make a shower gel that soothes you, wakes you up or just makes you smell good.

My son has a mild form of psoriasis and I find using cold tar based shampoos excellent for his scalp, so I add 25ml of this shampoo to 100ml of shower base so he can wash his whole body in it. This saves me money and it also saves him having to take both shampoo and soap to the rugby club.

I also have a penchant for a famous toiletries chain of shops shower gel which is quite expensive. However it is quite concentrated so, to make it go further, I dilute it 50 - 50 with a shower gel base and put it in another bottle.

You can also purchase baby shampoo fairly cheaply and make your own shower gels from that by adding essential oils to fragrance them. Baby shampoos are light and unscented which makes them the perfect base.

Bath gels are similar to shower gels and need diluting before use to help pouring and mixing with other ingredients. Again the manufacturer will provide dilution ratios for the bases. They also vary from basic bath gels to ones containing parabens, palm oils, sodium lauryl sulphate or organic bases and ones containing aloe vera or honey. You can buy liquid castile type soap fairly cheaply and this makes an excellent concentrated bubble bath.

Using these bases you can make specific washes that can help with different problems. The following recipes use 100ml of the diluted base and combinations of essential oils only. They can be made with shower or bath gel bases. Add the oils straight to the base in the bottle it is to be stored in and shake well.

Recipes Using Only Essential Oils

Refreshing

- 10 drops pine oil
- 10 drops sweet orange oil
- 8 drops juniper oil

Relaxing

- 12 drops lavender oil
- 8 drops neroli oil
- 8 drops geranium oil

Good Sleep

- 8 drops juniper oil
- 10 drops lavender oil
- 12 drops chamomile oil

Uplifting

- 10 drops geranium oil

- 8 drops jasmine oil
- 8 drops clary sage oil

Tension Reliever

- 10 drops lavender oil
- 10 drops melissa oil
- 8 drops bergamot oil

Balancing

- 10 drops lavender oil
- 10 drops geranium oil
- 8 drops patchouli oil

Winter Comfort

- 8 drops cypress oil
- 8 drops black pepper oil
- 8 drops sandalwood oil

Cold Relief

- 10 drops pine oil
- 8 drops eucalyptus oil
- 8 drops thyme oil

Warming

- 10 drops black pepper oil
- 6 drops ginger oil
- 10 drops frankincense oil

Ache Relief

- 10 drops basil oil
- 8 drops eucalyptus oil
- 8 drops lime oil

A Touch Of Luxury

- 10 drops rose oil
- 10 drops ylang ylang
- 10 drops frankincense oil

Adding Moisturisers And Other Beneficial Ingredients

Again the following recipes are based on using 100ml of shower or bath gel. These can be added along with the groups of essential oils in the above recipes to add to the effectiveness.

To Help Moisturise Normal Skin

Add 2 teaspoons of warmed honey to the base and shake well

To Help Moisturise Drier Skin

Add 1 teaspoon of olive oil, sweet almond or jojoba oil to the base and shake well each time you use it.

To Help Moisturise Very Dry Skin

Melt 2 teaspoons of cocoa butter or shea butter and mix it into the base

Toning

To tone the skin add 2 tablespoons of witch hazel to the base. Take this liquid into consideration when you dilute the concentrate.

Soothing

To calm irritation or over exposure to the sun, add 2 tablespoons of aloe vera gel to the base. This is excellent to take with you on holiday as you can make small amounts.

Extra Rich

Melt 2 teaspoons of cocoa butter, mix it with 2 teaspoons of sweet almond oil and 2 teaspoons of runny honey. Add to the base and shake well. The oils will separate on standing but will disperse when shaken before use.

10 FACIAL CLEANERS, TONERS, MOISTURISERS, SCRUBS AND MASKS

Cleansers, toners, scrubs and masks are very easy to make at home. True, moisturisers are a little more technical but they are still relatively easy to do.

Many of them use store cupboard ingredients but some require purposely bought ingredients like shea butter, cosmetic oils like sweet almond, coconut and apricot and obviously essential oils.

Other ingredients that are useful to have around are witch hazel, rose water (which you can make yourself - see chapter 9), beeswax, glycerine, creamed coconut and coconut milk powder.

The most important thing you have to remember about making home-made beauty products is that they will not contain any preservatives unless you add them. So make sure you store them in sterile containers and keep them securely lidded and in a dark, cool place. Use them up within a month and if you have an open sore of any kind on your face be extra careful about application to that area. Always use clean or sterilised implements to mix your products for extra safety and, if water is called for, always use cooled boiled water.

Cleansing

This is an important part of any beauty regime and simple yet effective home-made cleansers are easy to make.

Simple Cleansers

The following recipes make between 5 and 8 applications.

For Dry Skins

Method:

1.   Mix a small 5 pence sized amount of coconut oil with 2 drops of lavender oil (or frankincense oil for mature skins) and apply to the face.
2.   Massage all over avoiding the eye area.
3.   Wipe off with a soft face cloth dampened with warm to hot water.
4.   Repeat with the cloth, rinsing out 2 - 3 times. This is an efficient cleanser for removing make-up.

For Normal To Oily Skins

Method:

1.   Mix 2 tablespoons of cornflour with 500ml of cooled boiled water until smooth.
2.   Combine with 25ml of glycerine and heat in a bowl over a pan of boiling water.
3.   Stir well adding a little more boiled water to make a loose but not thin solution.
4.   When the mixture becomes transparent remove it from

the heat.

5.   Allow it to cool then stir in 5 drops of neroli or sweet orange oil for normal skins. For oily skins replace the neroli or sweet orange oil with 5 drops of thyme oil. If you have a tendency to break out in spots add 5 drops of tea tree oil.

6.   Apply the cleanser to the skin on a cotton wool pad and sweep over the face. This isn't very good at removing make-up - you would be best using an oilier one for this.

For Mildly Irritated Skin

Method:

1.   Mix 2 tablespoons of sweet almond oil, 1 tablespoon of witch hazel and 2 tablespoons of aloe vera gel in a clean lidded container.

2.   Cover and shake well.

3.   Use on a cotton wool pad and sweep over the face. This will remove surface dirt and most make-up types.

Other Cleansers That Require A Little More Preparation

Soothing Cleanser For All Skin Types

This makes about 5 - 6 applications.

Ingredients:

- 2 tablespoons oatmeal
- 50ml boiling water
- 2 tablespoons wheatgerm or sweet almond oil
- 2 tablespoons aloe vera gel
- 5 drops chamomile oil

Method:

1. Pour the boiling water over the oatmeal and stir well. Allow to cool and strain the liquid into a bottle or jar.
2. Add the other ingredients and cover with a lid. Shake well until everything is blended. If you prefer it slightly thicker add a little more oil.

To use apply to the skin with a cotton wool pad and massage in with the fingertips. Wipe off with a damp cotton wool pad.

Light Cleanser For Mature Skin

Makes 8 - 10 applications.

Ingredients:

- 4 tablespoons boiling water
- 1 tablespoon oatmeal
- 3 tablespoons glycerine
- 1 tablespoon wheatgerm or avocado oil
- 5 drops frankincense oil
- 5 drops rose oil
- 2 tablespoons rose water

Method:

1. Pour the boiling water over the oatmeal, cover and leave to steep.
2. Strain the liquid and pour into a bottle or jar.
3. Add all the other ingredients, cover and shake well.

Apply with the fingers or a cotton wool pad and remove with a warm damp face cloth.

This recipe is also good for dry skin. Use 5 drops of geranium oil in place of the frankincense oil to balance the skin.

For oily skin don't add the wheatgerm or avocado oil but add 5 drops of juniper oil or lemon oil in place of the geranium oil.

Toners

Toning the skin can be done simply by using cold water to splash onto the complexion after cleansing. There are other simple ways to tone your skin quickly. Pour some mineral oil into a pump action bottle and keep it in the fridge until needed, then spritz the face as necessary. Make it even more beneficial by adding 8 drops of lavender oil for normal to dry skin or 5 drops of rosemary oil and 5 drops of thyme oil for normal to oily skin.

Honey makes an excellent toner and is my favourite ingredient as it lightly moisturises, soothes and calms the skin as well as toning it.

Honey Water Toner

This can also be put into a pump action spray bottle or in an ordinary one with a good lid. Keep it in the fridge and shake well before you need to use it.

Ingredients:

- 100ml boiled water
- 2 tablespoons clear honey
- 5 drops cypress oil
- 5 drops geranium oil

Method:

1. Allow the boiling water to cool for a few minutes then mix into the honey.
2. Pour the honey mixture into a bottle and add the essential

oils.

3.   Shake well and apply to the skin when completely cool.

Use damp cotton wool pads to apply the toner to the facial and neck areas.

Cucumber Toner

This is good for refreshing normal to oily skins. You will need a square of cheesecloth and a sieve for this recipe.

Ingredients:

- 1 medium sized cucumber
- 2 teaspoons honey
- 1 tablespoon witch hazel

Method:

1.   Peel and chop the cucumber and place it in a food processor of blender. Purée until smooth and juicy.
2.   Place the sieve over a bowl and line it with the cheesecloth. Pour the cucumber purée into the sieve, cover it and leave it to drain through. It is the liquid you want for the toner. This process will take about 20 minutes.
3.   Pour the juice into a sterile bottle and add the honey and witch hazel. Put on the lid and shake well.

Apply to the skin with a damp cotton wool pad.

Carrot And Rosemary Toner

This is an excellent toner for calming spots and blemishes.

Ingredients:

- 50ml boiling water
- 1 tablespoon rosemary leaves
- 50ml carrot juice
- 5 drops rosemary oil

Method:

1. Pour the boiling water over the leaves and allow to steep until cold.
2. Strain the liquid and pour it into a prepared bottle.
3. Add the carrot juice and rosemary oil and shake well.

Apply to the skin with a cotton wool pad.

Witch Hazel And Lavender Toner

This is a good toner for all skin types and it has a light cleansing action.

Ingredients:

- 20ml distilled witch hazel
- 20ml cooled boiled water or lavender water
- 5 drops lavender oil

Method:

Combine all the ingredients in a prepared bottle and shake well before use.

A Gentle Toner For Mature Skins

This combines glycerine and rose water which are traditional cosmetic ingredients used throughout the centuries to enhance the complexion.

Method:

Stir 50ml each of rose water and glycerine together in a jug and pour into a sterile bottle. Add 5 drops of rose oil and 8 drops of frankincense oil. Put on the lid and shake well.

Moisturisers

Making your own facial moisturisers is a little more complicated but is well worth the effort. These ones will keep for a limited period - about 4 weeks - so only make them in small amounts.

Rich Facial Moisturiser

This makes about 50g.

Ingredients:

- 10g or a heaped teaspoon pure beeswax
- 2 tablespoons apricot kernel oil
- 2 tablespoons sweet almond oil or wheatgerm oil
- 2 rounded teaspoons shea butter
- 3 tablespoons rose water
- 5 drops rose oil

Method:

1.   Put the beeswax, oils and shea butter in a bowl over a

pan of very hot water and melt them together.

2.   Stir in the rose oil and beat in the rose water. The cream should become light and fluffy. If it is too stiff add more rose water. Store in a sterile, lidded jar.

Lighter Moisturising Cream

This is a lighter cream but it is still quite rich so a little goes a long way.

Ingredients:

- 20g coconut oil
- 20ml glycerine
- 10ml witch hazel
- 5 drops chamomile oil

Method:

1.   Melt the coconut oil in a bowl and beat in the glycerine, witch hazel and chamomile oil.
2.   Store in a sterile lidded pot.

Light Moisture Lotion

Ingredients:

- 3 tablespoons aloe vera
- 3 tablespoons glycerine
- 1 teaspoon sweet almond oil
- 5 drops camellia or melissa oil

Method:

1.   Put all the ingredients into a small bowl and beat them

together until light and fluffy.
2.   Store in a sterile lidded jar.

An easier way of preparing a moisturiser that suits your skin is to buy an aqueous lotion or cream from the chemist and add your own essential oils or other ingredients such as floral waters. They do contain mineral oils but can be purchased cheaply and are effective on dry skins.

Facial Masks

We're back in girly night in the city now. I love making these and dreaming up new ones. Many fruits can be used to help clean and tone the skin. Fruits have natural cleansers and exfoliants in them and so make excellent face packs, that is if you can stop yourself from eating them.

The only problem is that they can be a bit tricky to apply to the face and it can get very messy, so always protect your clothing. I prefer to apply them over the sink so any debris falls in there rather than on the carpet.

All the following masks make 1 application unless otherwise stated.

Make sure you only apply them to the facial area away from the eyes.

Banana Mask

This is an excellent conditioning mask for all skin types. It leaves the skin very soft and clean.

Ingredients:

- 1 ripe mashed banana
- 2 teaspoons sweet almond oil
- 1 teaspoon lemon juice
- 1 egg yolk

Method:

1.   Put the banana in a bowl and mix in the other ingredients thoroughly.
2.   Apply the mixture to the face then lie back and relax for

20 minutes.

3.   Remove with tissues and splash your face with cool water to finish.

Honey Mask

This not only helps firm the skin temporarily but brightens and softens it too.

Ingredients:

- 1 egg white
- 2 tablespoons honey
- 1 tablespoon finely ground oatmeal

Method:

1.   Whisk the egg white and add the other ingredients to form a paste.
2.   Apply to the face and leave for about 15 minutes. The mask will begin to dry out.
3.   Rinse off with cold water.

Apple And Honey Mask

This helps to liven up dull or tired skin.

Ingredients:

- 1 mashed or grated peeled apple
- 1 tablespoons clear honey
- 1 whole egg
- 1 tablespoon finely ground oatmeal

Method:

1. Put the apple and honey together in a bowl.
2. Beat the egg and stir it into the apple.
3. Add the honey and the oatmeal and stir well.
4. Apply to the face, massaging in gently.
5. Leave for 20 minutes then rinse off with cool water.

Avocado Mask

This is ideal for drier skin that needs a little tender loving care. It will also clean and soften the skin.

Ingredients:

- 1 avocado peeled and mashed
- 1 egg yolk
- 2 teaspoons apricot kernel oil
- 5 drops neroli oil

Method:

1. Put all the ingredients into a bowl and beat well together.
2. Apply to the skin and leave for at least 15 minutes (longer if you can stand it as it does slip about)
3. Remove with tissue and rinse with cool water.

Papaya Mask

This really brightens and cleans the skin effectively.

Ingredients:

- 4 tablespoons papaya flesh puréed or mashed
- 1 egg yolk

- 1 tablespoon natural yoghurt
- 5 drops grapefruit oil

Method:

1. Mix all the ingredients together in a bowl.
2. Apply to the skin and leave the mask on for 15 - 20 minutes and wipe off with tissues.
3. Splash the face with cool water to finish.

Strawberry Mask

This helps with blemishes that erupt now and again.

Ingredients:

- 6 - 8 ripe strawberries mashed well
- 1 tablespoon natural yoghurt
- 1 teaspoon lemon juice

Method:

1. Mix all the ingredients thoroughly in a bowl.
2. Apply to the face and leave for 15 - 20 minutes.
3. Remove with a tissue and splash the face with cool water.

Fuller's Earth Mask

This a deep cleansing mask that is good for oily skins. Fuller's Earth is a clay like substance that is used to cleanse oil or grease. It can be purchased from chemists.

Ingredients:

- 2 tablespoons Fuller's Earth
- 1 teaspoon lemon juice
- 2 teaspoons jojoba or sweet almond oil
- A little boiled water

Method:

1.   Put the fuller's earth in a bowl and add the lemon juice and oil.
2.   Mix to a smooth paste with the water and apply to the face.
3.   Allow to dry and rinse off with cool water.

Facial Scrubs

I use a facial scrub once a week as I think it keeps my skin looking healthy and bright. Making your own is just as good as buying expensive ones as they do exactly the same job. Even is you have sensitive skin there is something you can use to help keep your skin fresh and soft.

The best way to prepare the skin when you have cleansed it of dirt and make-up is to place a warm damp face cloth over your face for a few seconds before applying the scrub. This opens the pores ready to be cleansed.

Almond Scrub

This is a gentle scrub but it really works its way into the pores

Ingredients:

- 20g ground almonds
- 2 teaspoons sweet almond oil

- 5 drops geranium oil

Method:

1. Mix all the ingredients together and apply to the face, working in circular movements over the facial area. Again, avoid the eyes. Pay particular attention to the areas around the nose and chin.
2. Use a warm damp flannel to remove the scrub.

Coconut And Almond Scrub

This works well on dry skins and cleans and decongests the pores.

Ingredients:

- 20g ground almonds
- 1 teaspoon coconut oil
- 2 teaspoons desiccated coconut
- 5 drops geranium oil

Method:

1. Put everything in a bowl over a pan of hot water to melt the coconut oil and stir well.
2. When the coconut oil begins to set put it on your face and massage it in with circular movements.
3. Use a warm damp flannel to remove the debris and oil

Sugar Scrubs

For a more vigorous facial scrub I use caster sugar as I find granulated too coarse for my skin.

Ingredients:

- 2 tablespoons caster sugar
- 2 teaspoons olive oil
- A couple drops lavender, rosemary or geranium oil

Method:

1. Mix all the ingredients together in a bowl.
2. Dampen the skin and massage into the face with circular movements using your fingertips. The great thing about this is that when you wish to get rid of it it simply washes away with warm water. A warm damp face cloth will get rid of any excess oil. If you don't wish to use any oil, try a tablespoon of glycerine or aloe vera gel instead.

11 HANDS, FEET AND BODY TREATMENTS

This chapter covers all the parts of the body that at times need a little extra care like the knees, nails, hands and feet. Also scrubs for difficult areas like elbows, upper arms and heels.

Hands And Nails

I need to use a hand cream 2 - 3 times a day so I get through quite a lot of it. In the evening I like to use a rich hand cream that really does soften the dry skin around my forefingers and thumbs. This is where my skin cracks if I'm not careful. For a real deep down conditioning treatment I massage in my hand cream then put on some soft cotton gloves and wear them for an hour whilst I read or watch the television. This seems to do the trick even when my hands are very dry. I feel quite regal!

I buy shea butter for my nails and put a small amount in a little pot to massage into each nail every evening. This stimulate the circulation and helps nails stay strong and healthy. It seems to keep my cuticles soft as they used to crack and get sore. It has the added benefit of keeping my nails supple and stops them peeling or being brittle.

Another trick I learnt from my aunt was to massage a little olive oil onto your hands before putting on rubber gloves to do your washing up. The heat of the washing up water and the protection of the gloves intensifies the action of the oil on softening your hands.

Alternatively soak your hands in a bowl of warm water containing 2 tablespoons of glycerine and 8 drops of geranium oil. Have ready in a small container 1 tablespoon of almond, olive or sunflower oil and a warm towel. After you've soaked your hands for 5 minutes, massage in the oil when your hands are still damp and wrap them in the warm towel. You will have the softest hands ever.

Hate wearing gardening gloves? Scrape your fingernails along a bar of soap so that small bits get trapped under your nails. This stops dirt from accumulating there and, if any does, it is easily washed away with the soap.

Sugar Hand Scrub

When my hands are feeling particularly dry or uncomfortable I mix 1 tablespoon of olive oil with a rounded teaspoon of granulated sugar. I then gently massage the paste into my hands in a circular movement. Try it. I can promise that you will begin to feel a tingling sensation. Finally place your hands in warm water for a few seconds to dissolve the sugar, then pat them dry with a warm towel.

Rich Hand Cream

This is a rich hand cream you can easily make yourself. Store it in a sterile lidded jar and it will keep for up to 6 weeks.

Ingredients:

- 50ml apricot kernel oil
- 80g coconut oil
- 15g beeswax
- 2 teaspoons honey
- 1 vitamin E capsule or evening primrose capsule
- 2 tablespoons aloe vera gel
- 3 tablespoons rose water
- 10 drops lavender or rose oil

Method:

1.   Put the apricot and coconut oil and the beeswax in a bowl over a pan of hot water until they melt and stir them together.
2.   Add the honey and break open the capsule and stir into the beeswax mixture whilst it is still over the hot water.
3.   Mix the aloe vera with the rose water and essential oil
4.   Remove the bowl containing the beeswax mixture from the heat and when it has cooled slightly but it is still runny, beat in the aloe vera mixture until the whole thing is fluffy. This will firm up as it cools completely.
Transfer to the prepared jar while it is warm.

Nail Strengthening Hand Soak

Put sufficient warm water in a bowl to more than cover your hands. Then add 2 - 3 tablespoons of cider vinegar and 1 tablespoon of sweet almond oil. Leave your hands to soak in this for 5 - 8 minutes or until the water cools.

Hand and Nail Salve

This one is as good as the very famous hand salve by a big cosmetics firm.
Make sure you have a couple of clean lidded tins or containers

and store the finished product in a cool dark place.

Makes about 75g product

Ingredients:

- 50g beeswax
- 2 tbsp olive oil
- 2 tbsp coconut oil
- 1 tbsp sweet almond oil or apricot kernel oil
- 10 drops lavender essential oil
- 10 drops chamomile essential oil
- 8 drops tea tree essential oil

Method:

1. Place the beeswax, olive oil, coconut oil, and almond oil in a heatproof bowl.
2. Place over a pan of simmering water.
3. Stir gently until all the wax and oils are melted together.
4. Remove from the heat and stir in the 3 essential oils.
5. Pour into the lidded container and leave to cool and set.

The salve should be quite firm until you touch it, the warmth of your fingers will allow it to melt. Massage a little into your hands and nails. This is particularly effective if you treat your hands to a scrub beforehand.

A similar salve can be made to treat mature skins by adding evening primrose oil instead of the olive oil, replacing the tea tree essential oil with rosé oil and adding 10 drops of clary sage essential oil.

Nail and Cuticle Balm

This softens the cuticles and surrounding skin around the nails and strengthens the nail itself. Have ready some small lidded pots.

This makes about 30g of product

Ingredients:

- 25g Shea butter
- 1 dessertspoon sweet almond oil or wheat germ oil
- 12 drops lemon essential oil

Method:

1. Place all the ingredients in a small heat proof bowl and stand the bowl in hot water.
2. All the oils will melt into each other.
3. Stir gently, then pour into the containers.

Massage a tiny amount into each nail each evening, paying particular attention to the skin around the nail. Use daily when you need it or at least at night before going to bed. This gives the ingredients a chance to sink in overnight.

Hand Smoothing Mask

This softens and cleans your hands so it is particularly useful if you have been gardening. It lifts out grime and dead skin cells. Give yourself 30 minutes to allow this to work. It is a wonderful excuse to sit and relax and listen to some music as you won't be able to use your hands.

Ingredients:

- 1 tablespoon coconut milk powder
- 3 tablespoons hot water
- 2 tablespoons fine oatmeal
- 3 teaspoons sweet almond oil
- 5 drops juniper oil
- 5 drops lavender oil

Method:

1.   Mix the coconut milk powder and the hot water and add all the other ingredients to form a spreadable mixture. Add a little more warm water if necessary.
2.   Apply to the hands and massage in then leave to dry for as long as you can.
3.   Rinse off in warm water and apply a hand cream or lotion.

Fit Feet

Our poor feet get a real hammering what with our busy lives and being pushed into shoes and trainers. So much so that it is a real pleasure to give them some tender loving care at least once a week. My local beauticians do a wonderful deal on pedicures, but you can do the same at home at a fraction of the cost. The only difference is that you don't get someone else to massage your feet unless you have a friend or family member willing to do it. Just soaking your feet in warm water for 10 minutes makes all the difference, then massage in some cream or lotion.

Foot Soak Ideas

To Relax

- Stir 2 tablespoons epsom salts into warm water and add 15

drops lavender oil.

To Revive

- Stir 2 tablespoons sea salt and 10 drops eucalyptus oil into warm water. To warm - stir 2 tablespoons sea salt and 10 drops ginger oil into warm water.

To Eliminate Odour

- Stir in 2 tablespoons sodium bicarbonate and 10 drops cypress oil. To help with infections stir in 2 tablespoons sea salt, 10 drops tea tree oil and 10 drops lavender oil.

To Freshen

- Stir in 2 tablespoons sodium bicarbonate and 10 drops peppermint oil. After soaking and before drying, massage a little coconut oil into your feet and wrap in a warm towel. Leave for a few minutes until the towel has cooled down then pat them dry.

Foot Scrubs

Prior to soaking give your feet a scrub to get rid of the hard and dead skin and dead skin cells. Have a towel ready to rest your feet on and to collect the bits of scrub that fall off as you use it.

Sea Salt Scrub

Mix 3 tablespoons of coarse sea salt with 2 teaspoons of olive oil and 8 drops of neroli or sweet orange oil. Massage into the feet making sure you do around and in between the toes. This is also good for the knees.

Sugar And Honey Scrub

Mix 3 tablespoons of granulated sugar with 3 teaspoons of honey and 10 drops lemon oil. Mix everything together for a very sticky scrub. Have a bowl of warm water ready to plunge your sticky feet into. This really softens the skin and helps get rid of any hard skin that lingers around your heels.

This scrub is also good for your elbows and upper arms to get the circulation going and get rid of those stubborn lumps and bumps on the outer arm. After using a scrub on your elbows and upper arms, smooth on some aloe vera gel to moisturise and help with any blemishes. This also lessens the look of stretch marks around the upper arms.

Soothing Foot Balm

This is wonderful for tired and sore feet.

Have a bowl of warm water ready to rinse off the balm. Whilst the balm is working its magic, rest your feet on an old towel over a foot stool or something that raises your feet - this will help revive them as well.

Ingredients:

- 1 small pot natural yoghurt
- 1 tablespoon cider vinegar
- 2 tablespoons aloe vera gel
- 10 drops lavender oil

Method:

1.   Stir all the ingredients together and massage into your feet.
2.   Leave on for at least 10 minutes before rinsing off. Pat your feet dry with a soft warm towel.

Lips

When you wear make-up, but also as you get older, the lip line gets a little less defined and wrinkles start to appear, so much so that lipstick seems to find its way into those annoying lines. Ever since I started using a lip scrub followed by a balm I have found it has helped combat the onslaught of lines around my mouth area. Even if you don't wear make-up it is good to have softer lips, if for nothing other than just to pout.

I find a mild scrub helps keep my lips soft. After using a scrub a lip balm is just the thing to smooth over and keep your lips soft and protected from the elements.

Minty Scrub

Mix 1 teaspoon of caster sugar and a few drops of olive oil with a drop or two of peppermint oil and massage into the lip area for a few seconds before rinsing. The lips will tingle for a few minutes but once the circulation benefits from being stimulated they will be all soft and plumped up.

Oat Scrub

Mix 1 teaspoon each of ground almonds and fine oatmeal with a few drops of almond oil. Massage into the lip area for a few seconds before rinsing.

Rich Lip Balm

This is best stored in a small lidded pot. Keep it with you so you can apply it throughout the day. You can also add a little colouring if you wish.

This will make 2 small tubs of lip balm.

Ingredients:

- 15g beeswax
- 50ml sweet almond oil
- 10g shea butter
- 5 drops lemon oil

Method:

1. Put the beeswax, oil and shea butter together in a small bowl and heat over a pan of hot water until they melt and mix together.
2. Stir in the lemon oil and transfer to sterile lidded pots.

Apricot Oil Lip Balm

This is lighter than the previous recipe but still protects and softens the lips.

This makes 1 small pot full of balm.

Ingredients:

- 2 teaspoons beeswax
- 4 teaspoons apricot kernel oil
- 2 teaspoons shea butter
- 6 drops sweet orange essential oil

Method:

1.   Heat the wax, oil and butter together in a small bowl over a pan of hot water until everything melts and stir them together.
2.   Add the orange oil and stir and pour into the jar.

Simple Lip Balm

To make a quick and simple balm mix 2 teaspoons of aloe vera gel together with 2 teaspoons of warmed shea butter. This can be applied after the scrub and at nighttime. It helps with chapped and reddened lips that have been subjected to wintry weather as well.

Mouth Washes

After talking about the lips, let's stay in that area.

Here are some useful mouth wash recipes that are ideal for rinsing the mouth and refreshing the teeth and gums.

DO NOT SWALLOW ANY OF THE FOLLOWING MOUTH RINSES.

Minty Rinse

Makes 4 - 5 doses.

Ingredients:

- 100ml mineral water or cooled boiled water
- 10 drops peppermint oil

Method:

1. Combine the two ingredients in a bottle and shake well.

To Help With Sore Mouths

Mix 100ml of mineral or cooled boiled water with 15 drops of myrrh essential oil and use to rinse the mouth.

As A Gargle For Sore Throats

Mix 30ml of cooled boiled water with 5 drops of thyme oil and use to gargle with. Alternatively boil a teaspoon of fresh thyme leaves in 30ml of water for 2 - 3 minutes. Allow to cool completely. Strain and use the liquid to gargle with.

Toothpastes

These two recipes really do clean the teeth. Some recipes call for salt but just the very thought of it makes me feel sick. You can, however, add a teaspoon of salt to each of the following recipes if you feel so inclined.

Simple Minty Paste

Ingredients:

- 6 teaspoons baking soda
- 4 teaspoons glycerine
- 10 drops peppermint oil

Method:

1. Mix the ingredients together in a small pot. To use press a damp toothbrush in the paste and clean your teeth in the

normal way.

Deep Cleaning Toothpaste

Ingredients:

- 3 teaspoons arrowroot
- 3 teaspoons baking soda
- 3 teaspoons water
- 5 drops peppermint oil
- 3 drops clove oil

Method:

1. Mix all the ingredients together to make a smooth paste.
2. Press your damp toothbrush in the paste and use to clean the teeth in the normal way.

12 MAKING YOUR OWN TOILET WATER AND FRAGRANCES

Making your own floral waters, colognes and perfumed oils is much easier than you might think and whilst you are doing so it fills the house with wonderful aromas.

For your own safety, as with everything, always test anything you put on your skin on a small patch on your lower, inner arm just in case you are allergic to anything.

You can use any fragrant flowers for these recipes; lavender, rose petals, honeysuckle, lilac, rosemary, thyme, mint, calendula, sweet pea, freesia or perfumed apple blossom are some of the best. Try combining your favourites.

You will need to use distilled or de-ionised water in these recipes for the best and longest lasting results. Although water boiled for two minutes then cooled makes an easier way of diluting the fragrances, they won't keep as long.

Making Floral And Fragrant Waters

These were often made in households in the 18th and 19th

centuries and used to add fragrance to the hair and body.

You can use orange or any citrus peel and whole spices as well as flowers for this method. Gather flower heads or petals early in the day for the best results.

You will need:

- 2 identical heat proof bowls
- A large lidded pan that will hold the 2 bowls
- Distilled or de-ionised water
- About 2 medium sized tea cups of flower heads or petals
- Sterile bottles to store your water
- Lots of ice

Method:

1. Put the first bowl upside down in the pan and place the second bowl the right way up on top of it.
2. Put enough water in the pan to reach almost the top of the first bowl and then position the bowls so that they are in the centre of the pan.
3. Place the flowers in the water and then place on the heat to bring the water to the boil. Once boiled turn down the heat to a fast simmer and place the lid on upside down so the handle is facing into the top bowl.
4. Put the ice in the lid and as it melts get rid of it and replace it with new ice. The top bowl will gradually fill up with fragrant water. Keep an eye out for the bowl filling up and the water level not dropping too much.
5. When the bowl is almost full transfer it to the prepared bottles. This is best done using a funnel so that you don't waste any of the precious water.

This will keep fresh unopened for at least 4 months. Once opened use it within 2 weeks or 4 weeks if kept in the fridge.

Colognes

An excellent way of making your own cologne is by using distilled water and very high alcohol content vodka.

Combining Various Essential Oils You Can Create Your Own Personal Fragrance

I suggest that you get a good selection of essential oils. They are not cheap but you can buy them in small amounts and you only use a few drops at a time. I like to have lavender, ylang ylang, jasmine, rose, geranium, frankincense, lime, chamomile, lemon and sweet orange to hand.

You will need:

- 150ml distilled or de-ionised water
- 5 teaspoons vodka (as high an alcohol content as you can find)
- Essential oils of your choice
- A bottle to hold your fragrance (preferably a blue or brown glass bottle as this makes it keep for longer)

Method:

1.   Simply add everything to the bottle, put on the lid and shake well.

To test which smells go best together use a cotton wool bud for each fragrance and rub each smell onto a tissue to combine them and sniff. This way you only use tiny amounts and don't waste any of your precious oils.

Below are some of my favourite oil combinations but perfumes, as you know, are individual. Experiment and create your own 'signature' scent.

About 20 - 25 drops of essential oil gives a good dilution. Have fun giving your combinations names and don't forget to write down your favourite recipes.

- 10 drops lavender oil
- 5 drops lime oil
- 6 drops lemon oil

- 10 drops lavender oil
- 5 drops rose oil
- 6 drops chamomile oil

- 8 drops ylang ylang oil
- 6 drops jasmine oil
- 6 drops lavender oil

Making Your Own Essential Oils

The extraction of essential oils usually involves a distillation method using complicated equipment that enables the oil to be removed from the top of a liquid known as hydrosol. The liquid is also used as a cosmetic preparation, often as an after shave balm. The question is can it be done more simply at home without the use of elaborate tubes and pipes?

Yes it can. The finished product is not quite the same as a pure essential oil and nor is it as concentrated, but nevertheless you can make a very pleasant oil that can be used in the same was as a pure essential oil.

This method takes about 8 days to prepare but it is great fun and you get a real sense of achievement and well-being knowing you have made your own fragrant oil. My favourite is lavender as it produces a most pungent and long lasting fragrance. If you use rose petals use freshly picked ones from the most fragrant flowers you can find. Sweet peas give a wonderful result and though it isn't as strong as the lavender it is still worth having a go at. If you use freesia, use white or yellow ones as they seem to have the most concentrated perfume.

You will need:

- 150ml odourless vegetable oil such as olive oil, sweet almond or refined jojoba oil
- 4 lots of approximately 80g flower heads or petals freshly picked each time
- A sealable plastic bag
- A wide mouthed lidded jar (a Kilner jar is ideal)
- A rolling pin
- A cheesecloth or other means of filtering the flowers from the oil
- Lidded glass bottles for storing the oil (coloured ones are best and make sure they are sterile so the oil will store freshly)

Method:

1. Put the first lot of flowers into the plastic bag and expel as much of the air as possible. Seal it and bash the flowers with the rolling pin, bruising them well but not mashing them to a pulp.
2. Put the oil in a jar and mix in the bruised flowers. Put on the lid and keep it in a warm place for 2 days.
3. Repeat this process with the second lot of flowers using the same oil. Mix in the flowers well and seal. Leave for 2 days again.
4. Repeat this process with the other 2 lots of flowers.
5. After the final 2 days of leaving the flowers to infuse in the oil, strain the oil and pour it into the prepared bottles. Store them in a cool dark place and they should keep for 9

months to one year.

Use them to perfume your skin or in the bath as a luxurious soak.

An easy way to make a simple lavender or rose petal toilet water for immediate use is with a steamer. Place as many flowers as will fit into the top part of the steamer and steam them for about 30 minutes. Make sure you put sufficient water in the bottom pan to keep the mixture steaming. Allow it to cool with the flowers still in the top pan so that all the oils drop down into the base pan. Strain the mixture into a bottle when cool and keep it in the fridge. Use it within two weeks.

Citrus peel and spices can be used to make a winter fragrance. The whole of the house will smell gorgeous when preparing this.

To make life easier you can purchase an oil based ingredient called isopropyl myristate that is safe to use in perfume making. You can mix this with essential oils or concentrated fragranced oils to make your own perfumes. It gives an instant result. They will need a good shake each time you use them but it is very pleasant and light to use.

13 POTPOURRIS AND HOME FRAGRANCES

Potpourri in a book on making soap? Why? Well to me it seems an obvious connection as you will be using many of the same oils and can therefore make soap and a matching potpourri.

Potpourri has become very fashionable to have around the house. Many shops and stores stock the basic ingredients such as dried flowers and other natural items, fragrances and fancy dishes and bowls to contain them. There are many reasons to have them in strategic places around the home and the lounge, bathroom, stairs and landing seem to be the most popular. They don't just fragrance the air but can be used decoratively and adapted to fit in with your personal home décor. Potpourri is also useful for absorbing and getting rid of any unwanted odours as well as scenting the air. They can also be used seasonally to bring the outside space and atmosphere into the home. There are other ways to fragrance the home such as floral sachets, drawer liners and of course air fresheners and they will all contribute to a sweeter smelling home.

This is not however just a modern way of thinking. Historically herbs, flowers and spices have all been used and not just as air fresheners but also to protect against insect infestations and disease. Before moth balls were invented cotton sachets were made to hold dried and fresh herbs and flowers and hung up all around the house. In France and probably many other European countries lavender is still used on windowsills to stop insects from coming in through the open windows in summer.

So what are the benefits of making your own home fragrance enhancers? Well the biggest benefit, as with everything else you make yourself, is that you know precisely what has gone into it. Many commercially made potpourris contain dried ingredients and synthetic fragrances and many of these can cause irritation, especially if you have sensitive skin or chest problems. It is much cheaper too as you can use things from your own garden, walks in the forest or on the beach. The biggest cost will be the fragrances for which I would always recommend using natural essential oils. Mainly though it is fun to make it yourself and when you're out walking and find something that you can use in your potpourri it can be very exciting and will also serve to remind you of that particular walk or the place in which it was found.

Personally I have always found commercial air freshening sprays far too strong and as I have easily irritated sinuses I prefer not to spray chemicals around my house. So making your own comes down to common sense for both health reasons and your pocket.

Potpourri

Potpourri is easy to make but you will have to do a bit of planning about the ingredients. These are, however, easy to come by and you can use something as easy as flower petals.

Some Basic Natural Ingredients

- Flower petals, particularly brightly coloured and scented ones like calendula, rose, lavender, thyme and rosemary.
- Herb leaves such as thyme, rosemary, mint and lemon balm are good ones to grow for this.

- Whole spices like cinnamon, coriander, cloves, star anise, cardamom pods and allspice.
- Flower buds such as rose, mint blossom, lavender, rose geranium, chamomile and hops.
- Empty flower seed pods like poppy or honesty.
- Large seeds like sunflower or pumpkin.
- Whole flowers and small stems such as small marigolds, elderflower, cotoneaster or pyracantha stems which smell deliciously of honey and make an excellent inclusion in any potpourri.
- Fruit peels, particularly from citrus fruits, are particularly good for winter and Christmas mixtures.
- Pine and other fir cones, acorns, conker shells, nuts and nutshells, pussy willow, catkins and bits of bark, especially bits of bark that have resins on them as these are very fragrant.
- Beach debris such as shells, whelk cases, sea purses (actually dog fish egg cases) or any woody flotsam and jetsam.
- Leaves and certainly any herb leaf that you grow will be suitable for your potpourri and cat mint in particular has a very clean refreshing smell.
- Wood chips, particularly cedar wood and pine.
- Berries like juniper and hawthorn.
- Slices of fresh ginger root and pieces of mace.
- Whole or halved nutmegs.
- Moss and oak moss in particular as it holds fragrance well.

Many of these ingredients may be used straight away but some leaves and most flowers are better dried.

This can be done by placing them on a tray covered in two layers of good quality kitchen roll paper. Put the tray in a warm place away from moisture and condensation such as a dry airing cupboard or on top of a cupboard in the lounge. If you are drying any large flowers turn them every day so they dry evenly. Flowers and herbs may be dried in bunches and hung from ceilings.

When storing your ingredients keep them in air tight containers and, unless you don't mind the aromas combining beforehand, keep similar items together in separate jars.

Fixatives

When you are combining your ingredients together use an ingredient to fix the fragrance of the essential oils for the longest period of time. Use about 2 tablespoons of this fixative ingredient to about 10 tablespoons of other ingredients.

Here Are Some Fixative Ingredients Ideas

1. Chopped roots such as orris, calamus or sedge root.
2. Oak moss or other moss.
3. Wood chips.

Essential Oils To Fragrance Your Potpourri

Use pure essential oils and specifically those which are your favourites. Remember that any oil has its own unique qualities that can affect the mood or ambience of a room. Lavender and other calming oils like chamomile and clary sage are particularly good for bedrooms. Strong floral scents like rose, jasmine and ylang ylang are excellent in hallways and staircases. Citrus oils such as lemon, orange, grapefruit and my own favourite lime are good for bathrooms and kitchens.

When using these oils, and especially if you wish to mix them, put a small drop of each one to be used on a cotton wool pad and place it in a polythene bag. Leave it for a few seconds then have a good sniff to see if you like it. This way you can create just the right smell for the potpourri mix you have in mind. Always write down what you have used so that you don't forget the ingredients.

When combining fragrances in this way, use one essential oil to be your primary fragrance and no more than 3 others as accent scents. Twelve drops of the dominant smell to just 3 - 4 drops each of the others is about the correct amount for a medium sized bowl of potpourri, but more can be used if you like a pungent smell.

Combining The Ingredients

I think it is best to make it as freshly as possible, so make just the amount you need to fill each dish or bowl. Always use a glass or pottery container as plastic can deteriorate quickly when it comes into contact with essential oils.

Combine the ingredients together in a glass jar or a sturdy polythene bag and sprinkle them with your choice of essential oil. Shake the jar or bag to mix everything together and leave for 2 - 3 hours before pouring into the dish or bowl. You can leave the potpourri in a glass storage jar for weeks before using if you like. Remember you can also refresh your potpourri in this way after a few weeks or when it starts to lose its fragrance.

Some Favourite Recipes I Use

The following recipes are all named by me!

Spring Fresh

Ingredients:

- 2 tablespoons thyme leaves
- 2 tablespoons lemon balm leaves
- 2 tablespoons mint leaves
- 30 - 40g oak moss

- 5 small pine cones
- 12 drops rosemary oil
- 4 drops eucalyptus oil
- 4 drops lemon oil

Method:

1. Dry the leaves as described above for flowers for 3 - 4 days.
2. Break up the oak moss into small pieces.
3. Put everything in a polythene bag or glass jar and add the essential oils. Shake well and remove as much air as you can from the bag or jar. Tie it tight or secure the lid of the jar.
4. Leave it for 3 hours before transferring to a display dish or bowl.

Summer Floral

Ingredients:

- 2 tablespoons rose buds
- 2 elderflower heads
- 10 heads lavender flowers
- 1 tablespoon rose leaves
- 1 tablespoon rose geranium leaves
- 2 tablespoons rosewood chips
- 12 drops rose oil
- 4 drops lavender oil
- 4 drops palmarosa oil
- 4 drops geranium oil

Method:

1. Dry the flowers as described above for 3 days.
2. Mix with the rosewood chips and place in a bag or jar.

3.   Add the essential oils and shake well to mix.

4.   Secure the bag or lid on the jar and leave it for 3 hours before transferring to a display dish.

Christmas Special

Ingredients:

- The peel of 2 oranges
- The peel of 1 lemon
- 2 cinnamon sticks
- 10 whole cloves
- A small piece of ginger root sliced
- 2 tablespoons dried red rose buds
- 2 tablespoons cedar or pine wood chips
- 5 - 6 small pine cones
- 5 drops each of ginger, lemon and cinnamon oil

Method:

1.   Place the fruit peels and whole spices in a low oven at about gas mark ½, 140° C on a piece of baking paper on a baking sheet. If you cut them to the size you require beforehand they will certainly dry out quicker. Leave them for about 1½ hours then turn off the heat and leave for a further 2 hours or until dry.

2.   Break the cinnamon stick into 1cm pieces and mix with the other spices.

3.   Put all the ingredients together in a bag or jar and add the essential oils.

4.   Shake to mix well and secure the bag or the lid of the jar and leave for 3 hours before transferring to a display dish or a bowl.

Air Fresheners

Home-made air fresheners using essential oils can be not only deodorising but can also help to eliminate airborne bacteria and viruses. Using lavender, tea tree and other anti-viral/anti-bacterial oils is great if any family members have been unwell with tummy bugs, colds or flu. Never spray them too close to the face, however, and try not to inhale them too much.

How To Make An Air Freshener

What you will need:

- A large spray bottle
- 400ml cooled boiled water
- 25 drops lavender oil
- 20 drops tea tree oil
- 10 drops lemon oil
- 10 drops cypress oil

Method:

1. Pour the water into the spray bottle and add the oils. Replace the lid and shake well before each spraying.

In the summer when insects are a nuisance use 10 drops of citronella oil in place of the cypress oil.

For an uplifting air freshener add 20 drops of geranium oil in place of the tea tree and 10 drops of neroli oil in place of the lemon.

When colds and flu are in the air use 25 drops of lavender oil, 20 drops of lemon oil and 15 drops of eucalyptus oil as the essential oil recipe.

Drawer Liners

These are great for underwear and other smalls.

1. Use good quality wrapping paper but make sure the colour doesn't come off onto your things. Wall paper, in particular the unprinted type, is also good to use.
2. Simply cut the paper to fit into your drawer and place it on a flat, unpolished surface.
3. Fill a spray bottle with 50ml of water and 2ml of your chosen essential oil or combination of oils. Shake well and spray onto the paper. Don't saturate the paper too much or it may disintegrate or take ages to dry.
4. Hang it up to dry in a warm place (but not over a radiator) and leave it to dry completely before using it to line your drawer. You could also do the same with your favourite perfume if you wish.

Fragranced Sachets

These are something my aunt used to make as a young girl. She had them all over her house and would renew the dried flowers with fresh ones every year.

Use a muslin bag or home made small cotton bag to hold a large handful of dried lavender, rose petals and thyme or rosemary flowers. Any combination or any single flower can be used. Sprinkle with an appropriate essential oil and fill the sachet. Secure the top, preferably with a drawstring in a bow rather than a knot as knots are difficult to undo when you need to refill them. Hang these in wardrobes or over hangers or place them in your linen baskets or wherever materials of any sort are stored.